CW00497558

Therapeutic strength trainir

Karthikeyan Thangavelu

Therapeutic strength training for the treatment of spastic CP

Scholars' Press

Imprint

Any brand names and product names mentioned in this book are subject to trademark, brand or patent protection and are trademarks or registered trademarks of their respective holders. The use of brand names, product names, common names, trade names, product descriptions etc. even without a particular marking in this work is in no way to be construed to mean that such names may be regarded as unrestricted in respect of trademark and brand protection legislation and could thus be used by anyone.

Cover image: www.ingimage.com

Publisher:
Scholars' Press
is a trademark of
International Book Market Service Ltd., member of OmniScriptum Publishing Group
17 Meldrum Street, Beau Bassin 71504, Mauritius

Printed at: see last page
ISBN: 978-3-639-66138-5

Zugl. / Approved by: NIMHANS UNIVERSITY-2006

Copyright © Karthikeyan Thangavelu
Copyright © 2019 International Book Market Service Ltd., member of OmniScriptum Publishing Group

Dr.T.KARTHIKEYAN,MSPT,Ph.D.,D.LITT

Physiotherapist,

National Institute of Mental Health and Neuro Sciences, (NIMHANS)

(Institute of National Importance, A Government of India)

Bangalore-560029.

Karnataka,

India

ACKNOWLEDGEMENT

I am hearty thankful to Dr.Sekar (Registrar/DDA),

Dr.V.Bhadri Narayanan(HOD in physiotherapy unit) and

Dr. Anupam Gupta (Prof and HOD).

My sincere thanks to Prof. B.N.Gangadhar,

(Director & Vice-chancellor and Prof/ Dept of Psychiatry)

NIMHANS, and D.Nagaraja (Former Director & Vice-chancellor

Prof/Dept of Neurology)

NIMHANS, Bangalore for Last but encouraging me to do research work.

Dr.Shashidhar Buggi, Former Director, Professor and HOD

of CT Surgery,Rajiv Gandhi Institute of Chest Disease constant

encouraging me to do accomplishment of the research work.

I am thankful to me parents, my elder brothers, his wife,

his children and my brother in law and his wife (Er.I.Balamurugan).

Least I would like to thank all the subjects of my study,

without whom, this study would have not been possible.

T.KARTHIKEYAN

TOPICS

S.NO	CONTENTS	PAGE.NO
1.	Abstract	5-8
2.	Introduction	9-17
3.	Review of literature	18-20
4.	Methodology	21-33
5.	Data analysis	34-44
6.	Results	45
7.	Discussion	46-47
8.	Conclusion	48
9.	Limitations	49
10.	References	50-52

LIST OF ABBREVATIONS USED

CP   - Cerebral palsy

ROM   - Range of motion

ADL   - Activities of daily living

FSE   - First swing excursion

NoOS   - Number of Oscillations

DOS   - Duration of Oscillations

MD   - Mean deviation

SD   - Standard deviation.

M   - Mean

A STUDY TO ASSESS THE EFFECTS OF QUADRICEPS FEMORIS STRENGTHENING ON SPASTICITY IN CHILDREN WITH SPASTIC DIPLEGIC CEREBRAL PALSY

ABSTRACT

AIM OF THE STUDY

Background and Purpose: The Bobath neuro developmental treatment approach advised against the use of resistive exercise, as proponents felt that increased effort would increase spasticity. The purpose of this study was to test the premise that the performance of exercises with maximum efforts will increase spasticity in children with spastic diplegic cerebral palsy (CP).

OBJECTIVE OF THE STUDY

To study the effects of Quadriceps femoris strengthening on spasticity in children with spastic diplegic cerebral palsy.

HYPOTHESIS

Null Hypothesis:

Quadriceps femoris strengthening has no effect on spasticity in children with spastic diplegic cerebral palsy

Alternate Hypothesis:

Quadriceps femoris strengthening has effect on spasticity in children with spastic diplegic cerebral palsy

METHODOLOGY

SUBJECTS: Thirty children with spastic diplegic cerebral palsy ranging age from 5 to 8 years participated in a Quadriceps femoris strengthening program.

DURATION : 6 weeks

TREATMENT SESSION: - 3 Days/week

METHOD:

Knee muscle spasticity was assessed bilaterally using the pendulum test to elicit a stretch reflex immediately before and after different forms of Quadriceps femoris muscle exercise (isometric and isotonic) during a single bout of exercise training. Pendulum test outcome measures were: (1) first swing excursion, (2) number of lower leg oscillations and (3) duration of the oscillations. Pre test and post test was conducted.

STUDY SETTING:

Clinical set up study

STUDY DESIGN:

Quasi experimental study

STUDY SAMPLING:

Convenient sampling

SAMPLE SIZE:

30 Samples

SOURCE OF DATA:

NIMHANS Hospital, Bangalore

Study Duration:

Total duration was six weeks.

3 days per week

6

SAMPLING CRITERIAS

Inclusion Criteria:

- Diplegic spasticity
- Subjects of age of 5 to 8 yrs
- Good general health
- Ability to follow simple commands
- Ability to extend the knee from 90 to 45 in sitting position
- Not taking any pharmacological agent for reducing spasticity

Exclusion criteria:

- Subject below 5 and above 8 yrs of age
- Hip flexor tightness
- Hip adductor tightness
- TA tightness
- Fractures of Hip and knee
- Pain or orthopaedic problems affecting the legs
- Unstable seizures

Materials used:

Couch, goniometre, pendulum exercise. towel, etc..

DATA ANALYSIS:

The pre and post test data has been collected from the subjects. The data has to be analyzed in statistics using the paired t test and simple t test.

RESULTS

There were changes in spasticity following Quadriceps femoris strengthening exercise . i.e spasticty has not increased after Quadriceps femoris strengthening exercise .

CONCLUSION

The results do not support the premise that exercises with maximum efforts increase spasticity in children with spastic diplegic cerebral palsy.

INTRODUCTION

Cerebral Palsy is considered a neurological disorder caused by a non-progressive brain injury or malformation that occurs while the child's brain is under development. Cerebral palsy (CP) is defined as a clinical syndrome characterized by a persistent disorder of posture or movement due to a non-progressive disorder of the immature brain.

The prevalence of cerebral palsy is 2 to 2.5 per 1,000 live births and its incidence may be increasing secondary to improved care in neonatal intensive care units and improved survival of low birth-weight infant. Most children with CP will have spasticity as the main motor disorder.

It can be classified either according to which body areas is affected: hemiplegia, diplegia, tetraplegia, or the movement disorder type: spastic, athetoid, ataxic and hypotonic cerebral palsy

Spasticity in children can result from any disease process that affects the upper motor neuron within the central nervous system. Spasticity is a major challenge for rehabilitation of children with cerebral palsy. Spasticity is defined as a velocity dependent increased resistance to passive muscle stretch, or alternatively as inappropriate involuntary muscle activity associated with upper motor neuron paralysis. Spasticity can result in functional problems with daily living activities (ADL) such as gait, feeding, washing, toileting and dressing.

Spastic cerebral palsy is caused by damage to the motor cortex and the pyramidal tracts of the brain, which connect the motor cortex to the spinal cord. Understanding the function of the motor cortex and pyramidal tracts helps to explain how damage to these systems affects movement in those with spastic cerebral palsy.

Damage to the Motor Cortex

The motor cortex is located in the cerebral cortex, which is the largest part of the brain. The motor cortex is composed of several parts that are responsible for relaying signals to other parts of the brain to control movement.

The most important aspect of the motor cortex in relation to cerebral palsy is its regulation of voluntary movement. Damage to this region of the brain makes voluntary movement harder to control and less fluid, or "spastic".

Damage to the Pyramidal Tracts

The pyramidal tracts in the brain are the roads of communication between the cerebral cortex and the nerves in the spinal cord. If pyramidal tracts are damaged, the motor cortex can't send proper signals to the spinal cord. The spinal cord is one half of the central nervous system, with the other half being the brain and brain stem. These parts of the brain are essential for sensory functions such as sight, touch and movement.

The motor cortex and pyramidal tracts may be damaged by:

  - ➤ Prenatal brain hemorrhage or infection
  - ➤ Lack of oxygen to the brain during birth
  - ➤ Brain trauma or infection after birth

Over time, spasticity may also cause problems, such as muscle pain or spasms, trouble moving in bed, difficulty with transfers, poor seating position, impaired ability to stand and walk, dystonic posturing muscle, contracture leading to joint deformity, bony deformation, joint subluxation or dislocation and diminished functional independence.

Muscle strengthening as a treatment intervention has gained in popularity in the past 10 years since earlier concerns that strengthening would increase spasticity and produce abnormal movement patterns appear unfounded. This review critically analyses the current literature to determine the evidence of the effectiveness of muscle strengthening in children with cerebral palsy. It is reassuring to see that in more recent years there has been an increase in the quality of studies performed to examine the effects of strengthening in children with cerebral palsy.

CLASSIFICATION OF CEREBRAL PALSY

Cerebral Palsy: Topographic

* Monoplegic
* Hemiplegic
* Quadraplegic
* Diplegic

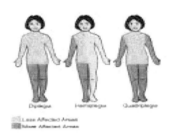

Figure:1

TYPES OF CEREBRAL PALSY

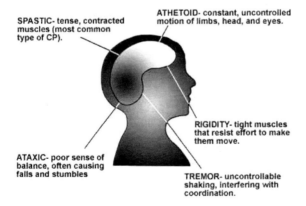

SPASTIC- tense, contracted muscles (most common type of CP).

ATHETOID- constant, uncontrolled motion of limbs, head, and eyes.

RIGIDITY- tight muscles that resist effort to make them move.

ATAXIC- poor sense of balance, often causing falls and stumbles

TREMOR- uncontrollable shaking, interfering with coordination.

Figure:2

AIM OF THE STUDY

The aim of this Study is to test the premise that the performance of Quadriceps femoris strengthening exercises with maximum efforts will increase spasticity in children with spastic diplegic cerebral palsy (CP).

NEED FOR THE STUDY

Cerebral palsy related to genetic abnormalities cannot be prevented, but however it is, a few of the risk factors for congenital cerebral palsy can be managed or avoided. One of the major risk factor is the spasticity. The Bobath neuro developmental treatment approach advised against the use of resistive exercise, as proponents felt that increased effort would increase spasticity. The purpose of this study was to test the premise that the performance of Quadriceps femoris strengthening exercises with maximum efforts will increase spasticity in children with cerebral palsy (CP) and this study could further pave the way for future research.

OBJECTIVE OF THE STUDY

The objective of this study is to test the premise that the performance of Quadriceps femoris strengthening exercises with maximum efforts will increase spasticity in children with cerebral palsy (CP).

HYPOTHESIS

Null hypothesis Ho:

Quadriceps femoris strengthening exercise has no effect on spasticity in children with cerebral palsy.

Alternate Hypothesis H1:

Quadriceps femoris strengthening has effect on spasticity in children with spastic diplegic cerebral palsy

OPERATIONAL DEFINITIONS

Cerebral Palsy:

Cerebral Palsy (CP) is a disorder of movement and posture that appears during infancy or early childhood. It is caused by non progressive damage to the brain before, during, or shortly after birth. CP is not a single disease but a name given to a wide variety of static neuro motor impairment syndromes occurring secondary to a lesion in the developing brain. The damage to the brain is permanent and cannot be cured but the consequences can be minimized. Progressive musculoskeletal pathology occurs in most affected children.

Spasticity :

Spasticity (from Greek *spasmos-*, meaning "drawing, pulling") is a feature of altered skeletal muscle performance with a combination of paralysis, increased tendon reflex activity and hypertonia. It is also colloquially referred to as an unusual "tightness", stiffness, or "pull" of muscles.

Clinically, spasticity results from the loss of inhibition of motor neurons, causing excessive velocity-dependent muscle contraction. This ultimately leads to hyperreflexia, an exaggerated deep tendon reflex. Spasticity is often treated with the drug baclofen, which acts as an agonist at GABA receptors, which are inhibitory.

Spastic cerebral palsy:

Spastic cerebral palsy is the most common type of cerebral palsy. The muscles of people with spastic cerebral palsy feel stiff and their movements may look stiff and jerky. Spasticity is a form of hypertonia, or increased muscle tone. This results in stiff muscles which can make movement difficult or even impossible.

Isometric quadriceps exercises:

Isometric quadriceps exercises aim to strengthen the quads by contracting the muscle, with no or very little movement of the knee joint. They are ideal exercises for early stage rehab to prevent muscle wasting.

Isotonic exercise:

Isotonic Exercise when a contracting muscle shortens against a constant load, as when lifting a weight. Isotonic exercise is one method of muscular exercise. In contrast, isometric exercise is when muscular contractions occur without movement of the involved parts of the body.

The first swing excursion:

The first swing excursion was the best predictor of the degree of spasticity in persons with CP. It is the first of the knee joint extension.

Number of oscillations:

It is the number of times which the cerebral palsy child is able to perform the oscillations.

Duration of oscillations:

It is the time taken for the number of oscillations which the cp child is able to perform.

REVIEW OF LITERATURE

Cerebral palsy (CP) is an unprogressive chronic encephalopathy that leads to neurological disorder (SCHOLTES, DALLMEIJER, RAMECKERS ET AL., 2008; SCHOEN, RICCI AND OLIVEIRA, 2003; DAMIANO, DODD AND TAYLOR, 2002; DARRAH, WESSEL, NEARINGBURG ET AL., 1999).

There are many different types of cerebral palsy, with spastic cerebral palsy being the most common (Lehman et al., 2008).

The study by Andersson et al. (2003) examined mobility in adults with cerebral palsy, and spasticity as well.

Spasticity as a velocity-dependent hyperexcitability of the muscle stretch reflex, consistent with the definition proposed by Lance in 1980

Spastic diplegia is highly prevalent in CP (SCHOEN,RICCI AND OLIVEIRA, 2003; SOUZA AND FERRARETO, 1998) whereby about 70% of children with diplegia have bilateral spasticity compromising the motor control of lower limbs, thougth they are able to walk.

Literature reviews have shown that the restrict capacity to generate force is as debilitating or more than it is the muscle spasticity, potentially causing more restriction to the movement than the spasticity itself (ROSS AND ENGSBERG,2007;SCHOLTES, DALLMEIJER, RAMECKERS ET AL., 2008).

Minimizing the harmful effects of spasticity has been the rehabilitation focus for these patients (FLETT, 2003; NORDMARK, JARNLO and HAGGLUND, 2000)

The progressive loss of the muscle strength, as this, together with spasticity, interferes directly with the motor rehabilitation strategies (SCHOLTES, DALLMEIJER, RAMECKERS et al., 2008; ROSS and ENGSBERG, 2007; DAMIANO and ABEL, 1998).

Damiano and Abel (1998) reported that in spite of fundamental importance in the normal motor control, the deficiencies of strength in the cerebral palsy child and the respective correlations with the motor capacity have been little investigated.

Studies have shown the benefits of strengthening exercises applied on CP patients. Isotonic, isometric, and isokinetic exercises have been utilized to faster increasing muscle strength and improvement of the motor function (BERRY, GIULIANI and DAMIANO, 2004; DAMIANO, KELLY and VAUGHN, 1995; FOWLER, HO, NWIGWE et al., 2001).

Dr. Karel Bobath and Dr. Berta Bobath developed a theory in the 1940's suggesting that strengthening a spastic muscle would increase the contraction, thus increasing the spasticity
.

Ross and Engsberg, on the other hand, discovered that there was no correlation between strength and spasticity

Fowler et al. (2001) specifically examined whether or not performance of exercises with maximum efforts would increase spasticity in people with cerebral palsy. Twenty-four participants with cerebral palsy performed three different forms of quadriceps femoris exercises (isometric, isotonic, and isokinetic). Knee spasticity was measured bilaterally immediately before and after the exercises using the pendulum test to obtain a stretch reflex. The measurements taken by Electrogoniometers in the Pendulum test included the first swing excursion, number of lower leg oscillations, and duration of the oscillations. The results of the study showed no increase in quadriceps femoris spasticity after maximum efforts.

The pendulum test, first described by Wartenberg, involves lifting the relaxed leg against gravity and releasing it, causing it to swing freely. The pendulum test has been reported to yield reliable measurements and to be sensitive to variation in spasticity in people with CP.

Bohannon assessed the reliability of measurements obtained with the pendulum test in people without known neurological impairments to quantify knee joint motion

ANDERSSON ET AL. (2003) examined the effects of progressive strength training on seven individuals with cerebral palsy

SALEM & GODWIN examined ten children with cerebral palsy to assess mobility after task-oriented strength training. Five children were assigned to the experimental group, and five were in the control group. The children placed in the experimental group received task-oriented resistance training focusing on lower body strengthening, while the children in the control group focused on improving balance through reinforcement and normalization of movement patterns through conventional physical therapy (Salem & Godwin). Mobility was measured using the Gross Motor Function Measure and the Timed "Up and Go" test.

BLUNDELL ET AL. (2003) examined eight children between the ages of four and eight, with cerebral palsy, who participated in a training program that lasted four weeks. The participants underwent exercises that were similar to daily tasks in order to increase functional ability.

JAN S.TECKLIN (2002) Strengthening training program can be used with children as young 5to 9 years. For the therapist to develop a training program, the child must be able to lift a load two or three times before fatigue in order to strengthen the muscles.

NYSTROM EEK ET AL. (2008) investigated the influence of strength training on gait in children with cerebral palsy.

DODD, K.J., TAYLOR, N.F., & GRAHAM, H.K. (2003), *Developmental Medicine & Child Neurology,* 45, 652-657. Strength training in young people with cerebral palsy concluded that the evidence supports strength training for increasing strength in children with CP without increasing spasticity or muscle tightness[14]

AN ELECTRONIC SEARCH was performed in May 2008 of the following databases: MEDLINE, Embase, CINAHL, PubMed, Database of Reviews of Effectiveness (DARE), the Physiotherapy Evidence Database (PEDro), and Cochrane Database of Systematic Reviews. Keywords used in the search included 'cerebral palsy', 'treatment outcome', 'physical therapy (specialty)/or physical therapy modalities/ or physiotherapy'. The Oxford Centre for Evidence-based Medicine Levels of Evidence (May 2001) were used to assign a level of evidence for each study

The current evidence for strengthening suggests that targeted strength training can improve the strength of particular muscle groups for children with CP in GMFCS levels I-III as measured at the body function and structure level without provoking increases in spasticity.

DESIGN AND METHODOLOGY

STUDY DESIGN

A Quasi experimental study design was conducted.

SAMPLE SIZE

30 individuals who fulfilled the inclusion and exclusion criteria were selected.

SAMPLE DESIGN

Convenient Sample

STUDY SET UP

Paediatric Therapy centre, NIMHANS

STUDY DURATION

Total duration was six weeks.

3 days per week

VARIABLES

Dependent variables: Spasticity of Lower limb

Independent variable: Quadriceps strengthening Exercise

SAMPLING CRITERIAS

Inclusion Criteria:

- Diplegic spasticity
- Subjects of age of 5 to 10 yrs
- Ability to follow simple commands
- Good trunk control
- Good Hip control
- Quadriceps weakness

Exclusion criteria:

- Subject below 2 yrs of age
- Hip flexor tightness
- Hip adductor tightness
- TA tightness
- Fractures of Hip and knee
- Pain or orthopaedic problems affecting the legs
- Unstable seizures

MEASUREMENT TOOLS

The measurement tools used are:

1. First swing excursion
2. Number of Lower leg oscillations
3. Duration of oscillations

MATERIALS USED

COUCH

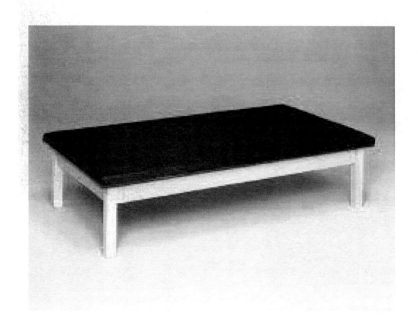

Figure :3

GONIOMETRE

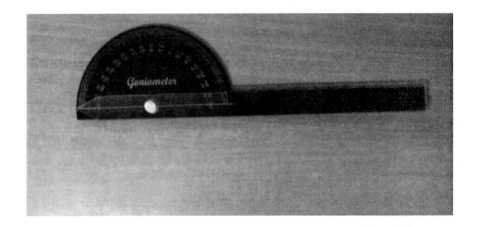

Figure :4

PILLOW

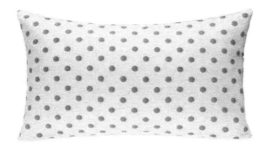

Figure :5

STOP WATCH

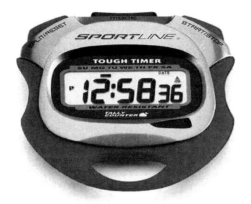

Figure :6

TOWEL

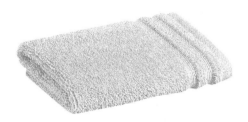

Figure :7

METHOD

Knee muscle spasticity was assessed bilaterally using the pendulum test to elicit a stretch reflex immediately before and after 3 different forms of right Quadriceps femoris muscle exercise (isometric, isotonic) during a single bout of exercise training. Pendulum test outcome measures were: (1) first swing excursion, (2) number of lower leg oscillations, and (3) duration of the oscillations.

Quadriceps strengthening exercises

Isometric quadriceps exercises aim to strengthen the quadriceps by contracting the muscle, with no, or very little movement of the knee joint. They are ideal exercises for early stage rehab to prevent muscle wasting.

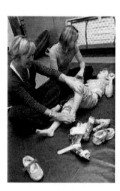

Figure :8

a) **Static quadriceps** – Patient is made to sit in the long seated position with back support. Due to quadriceps weakness knee will be in slight flexion. The patient is asked to press the knee against the floor up to the maximum limit of straightening the knee maintaining the foot in neutral positions.

b) **Dynamic quadriceps strengthening** – The patient is made to sit on a high sitting chair with the legs dangling with knee in 90 degree flexion initially without weight bring the knee into 90 degree extension or the maximum extension range possible from 90 degree knee flexion. Once the patient is able to do and maintain the knee in full extension without weight then gradually repeat the exercise with gradual increase in weight, depending on the age and capacity of the patient.

c) **Squats-** The patient is made to stand with bilateral weight bearing with or without support with maintaining the heel in neutral position, the patient is made to squat down then gradually come up with extending the knee up to the maximum limit.

Goniometric Measurement

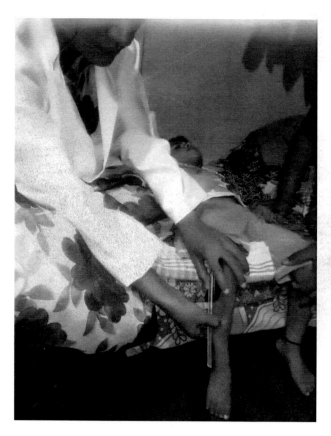

Figure: 9

Quadriceps Isometric Exercise

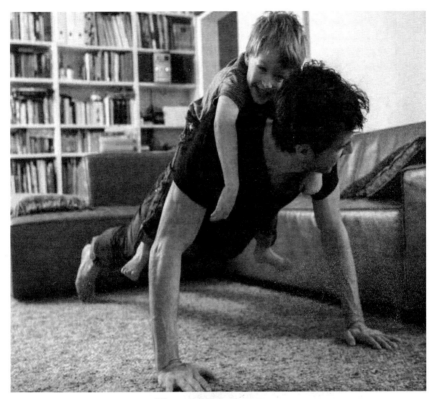

Figure :10

Isotonic Exercise

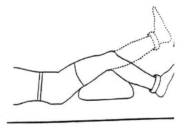

Figure: 11

STATISTICAL METHODOLOGY

Intra-Group Analysis (Within Group Analysis)

Objective:

To study the effect of Quadriceps strengthening Exercise (both "Isometric Exercise" and "Isotonic Exercise") in improving various measures such as FSE, NoOS, and DOS on left and right side.

Hypothesis:

Null Hypothesis, H_0: $\mu_d = 0$
(i.e., there is no significant effect of treatments in improving FSE/NoOS/DOS)

Alternate Hypothesis, H_1: $\mu_d > 0$ or $\mu_d < 0$ (*One-tailed test*)
(i.e., there is significant effect of treatments in improving FSE/NoOS/DOS)

In this case, μ_d = mean difference in scores between Pre and Post treatment;
d = difference ➔ d = Post Test Score – Pre Test Score

Level of significance, $\alpha = 0.05$

Test to be applied: Paired Sample t-test

Test Statistic: $t = \dfrac{\mu_d - 0}{s_d / \sqrt{n}}$

DATA ANALYSIS

1. FSE – Right Side

Testing the Pre and Post-test scores of FSE – Right Side using Paired t-test and the corresponding output is shown below:

t-Test: Paired Two Sample for Means-FSE-Right side

t-Test: Paired Two Sample for Means

	FSE_R2	FSE_R1
Mean	78.0417	77.1667
Variance	11.7143	10.9548
SD	3.4226	3.3098
Observations	60	60
Pearson Correlation	0.9824	
Hypothesized Mean Difference	0	
Df	59	
t Stat	10.5583	
P(T<=t) one-tail	0.0000	
t Critical one-tail	1.6711	
P(T<=t) two-tail	0.0000	
t Critical two-tail	2.0010	

Table: 1

Result: There is significant improvement in FSEon rightside due to the treatment ($t = 10.56$, $p < 0.05$). The mean value of FSE-right side is increased from 77.17 (SD = 3.31) to 78.04 (SD = 3.42) and this improvement is visually presented as follows:

Mean First Swing Excursion - Right Side

Pre & Post Test

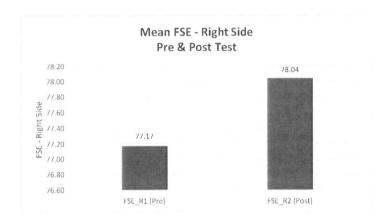

Mean FSE - Right Side
Pre & Post Test

Graph : 1

2. NoOS – Right Side

Testing the Pre and Post-test scores of NoOS – Right Side using Paired t-test and the corresponding output is shown below:

t-Test: Paired Two Sample for Means -NoOS Right side

t-Test: Paired Two Sample for Means

	NoOS_R2 (Post)	NoOS_R1(Pre)
Mean	4.6667	3.9333
Variance	0.4209	0.2582
SD	0.6488	0.5081
Observations	60	60
Pearson Correlation	0.6255	
Hypothesized Mean Difference	0	
Df	59	
t Stat	11.0000	
P(T<=t) one-tail	0.0000	
t Critical one-tail	1.6711	
P(T<=t) two-tail	0.0000	
t Critical two-tail	2.0010	

Table: 2

Result: There is significant improvement in NoOS on right side due to the treatment ($t = 11.00$, $p < 0.05$). The mean value of NoOS-right side is increased from 3.93 (SD = 0.51) to 4.67 (SD = 0.65) and this improvement is visually presented as follows:

36

Mean Number of Lower leg Oscillations- Right Side

Pre & Post Test

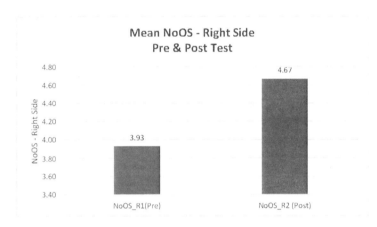

Graph: 2

3. DOS – Right Side

Testing the Pre and Post-test scores of DOS – Right Side using Paired t-test and the corresponding output is shown below:

t-Test: Paired Two Sample for Means -DOS Right side

t-Test: Paired Two Sample for Means

	DOS_R2 (Post)	DOS_R1 (Pre)
Mean	3.2500	3.2567
Variance	0.1653	0.2981
SD	0.4065	0.5460
Observations	60	60
Pearson Correlation	0.7369	
Hypothesized Mean Difference	0	
Df	59	
t Stat	-0.1399	
P(T<=t) one-tail	0.4446	
t Critical one-tail	1.6711	
P(T<=t) two-tail	0.8892	
t Critical two-tail	2.0010	

Table:3

Result: There is no significant change in DOS on right side due to the treatment ($t = -0.1399$, $p = 0.4446 > 0.05$). The mean value of DOS-right side before (Mean = 3.26, SD = 0.55) and after (Mean=3.25, SD = 0.41) the treatment is approximately same (i.e., Mean ≈ 3.3).

4. FSE – Left Side

Testing the Pre and Post-test scores of FSE – Left Side using Paired t-test and the corresponding output is shown below:

t-Test: Paired Two Sample for Means- FSE- Left side

t-Test: Paired Two Sample for Means

	FSE_L2(Post)	FSE_L1 (Pre)
Mean	78.0000	77.1667
Variance	11.1186	11.1921
SD	3.3345	3.3455
Observations	60	60
Pearson Correlation	0.9861	
Hypothesized Mean Difference	0	
Df	59	
t Stat	11.5798	
P(T<=t) one-tail	0.0000	
t Critical one-tail	1.6711	
P(T<=t) two-tail	0.0000	
t Critical two-tail	2.0010	

Table: 4

Result: There is significant improvement in FSEon left-side due to the treatment ($t = 11.58$, $p < 0.05$). The mean value of FSE on left-side is increased from 77.17 (SD = 3.34) to 78.00 (SD = 3.34) and this improvement is visually presented as follows:

39

Mean First Swing Excursion – Left Side

Pre & Post Test

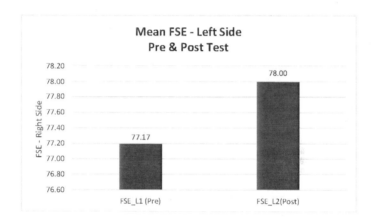

Graph: 3

5. NoOS – Left Side

Testing the Pre and Post-test scores of NoOS – Left Side using Paired t-test and the corresponding output is shown below:

t-Test: Paired Two Sample for Means- NoOS-Left side

t-Test: Paired Two Sample for Means

	NoOS_L2 (Post)	NoOS_L1 (Pre)
Mean	4.9667	4.3000
Variance	0.7446	0.5525
SD	0.8629	0.7433
Observations	60	60
Pearson Correlation	0.5179	
Hypothesized Mean Difference	0	
Df	59	
t Stat	6.4918	
P(T<=t) one-tail	0.0000	
t Critical one-tail	1.6711	
P(T<=t) two-tail	0.0000	
t Critical two-tail	2.0010	

Table: 5

Result: There is significant improvement in NoOSon left-side due to the treatment ($t = 6.49$, $p < 0.05$). The mean value of NoOS on left-side is increased from 4.30 (SD = 0.74) to 4.97 (SD = 0.86) and this improvement is visually presented as follows:

Mean Number of Oscillations - Left Side

Pre & Post Test

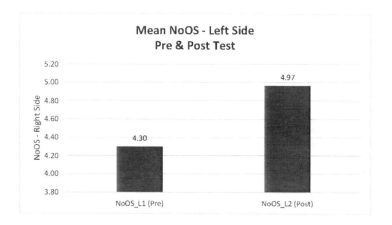

Graph: 4

6. DOS – Left Side

Testing the Pre and Post-test scores of DOS – Left Side using Paired t-test and the corresponding output is shown below:

t-Test: Paired Two Sample for Means-DOS- Left side

t-Test: Paired Two Sample for Means

	DOS_L2 (Post)	DOS_L1 (Pre)
Mean	3.1667	3.1667
Variance	0.1243	0.1243
SD	0.3526	0.3526
Observations	60	60
Pearson Correlation	1.0000	
Hypothesized Mean Difference	0	
Df	59	
t Stat	#DIV/0!	
P(T<=t) one-tail	#DIV/0!	
t Critical one-tail	#DIV/0!	
P(T<=t) two-tail	#DIV/0!	
t Critical two-tail	#DIV/0!	

Table:6

Result: The mean value (3.1667) and standard deviation (0.3526) of DOS on left-side are appears to be same before and after the treatment, due to which the Paired t-test cannot be performed for this data. This suggests that there is no significant change in the score of DOS left- side due to the treatment.

Mean Duration of Oscillations – Left side

Pre test and Post test

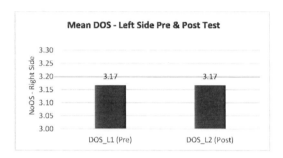

Graph : 5

RESULTS

From the above results, we see that on both left and right-side, there is significant improvement in FSE and NoOS values, while there is no significant change in the value of DOS due to the effect of Quadriceps strengthening on spasticity in children with spastic diplegic cerebral palsy.

DISCUSSION

A fundamental problem in the interpretation and application of Bobath concepts is that their clinical view of "spasticity" differs substantially from the definition that is widely adopted and supported today. The Bobaths described spasticity as a phenomenon that could be assessed by observing a patient move. They stated that hypertonus is caused by tonic reflexes (tonic labyrinthine, asymmetrical tonic neck reflexes; symmetrical tonic neck reflexes; associated reactions; and positive and negative supporting reactions), and they included co-contraction and "abnormal coordination" in their description of spasticity. They were critical of clinicians who measured spasticity at the "local muscular" level. Clearly, their descriptions differed from the definition accepted by neuroscientists in 1980 and used for the present study. In this definition, spasticity is a velocity-dependent increase in muscle stretch reflexes resulting from hyperexcitability of the stretch reflex, as one component of the upper motor neuron syndrome.

Children with CP did not demonstrate a greater difference in quadriceps femoris muscle spasticity immediately following strengthening exercises. Thesis finding refutes the premise that the performance of exercises with maximum efforts will result in a large, or detrimental, increase in spasticity. The maximum possible change in spasticity in either direction was substantially less than the change that was believed to create a clinically perceptible change. Confidence intervals are a means of providing insight into the maximum difference that would be likely if there were a large subject population . Confidence intervals was less than 0.05 which proved the effectiveness of improvement in the treatment in post test.

The considerable variation in spasticity within the group of subjects with CP was a potential confounding variable that could have been masked in the ANOVA. We recruited a greater number of subjects with CP and created subgroups based on severity of spasticity, and the statistical tests performed did not result in significant findings. These groups, however, were not equal and contained a small number of subjects. Despite these limitations, we believe that the severity of spasticity was not an important factor. The change in mean first joint excursion following exercise, our most sensitive measure was slightly greater for subjects with CP and no detectable quadriceps femoris muscle spasticity was detected.

The Thesis was started with the intention to refute the premise that Quadriceps strengthening increases spasticity. The two hypothesis stated in the thesis are Null Hypothesis and alternate Hypothesis.

The Null Hypothesis stated that there is no significant change in spasticity before and after Quadriceps strengthening which means that the spasticity remains the same without any increase or decrease before and after Quadriceps strengthening. However it is, the null hypothesis was rejected in the study.

The second hypothesis, alternate hypothesis which was stated as there is significant change in spasticity before and after Quadriceps strengthening which indicates that there is improvement in Quadriceps strengthening which has led to slight decrease in spasticity.

46

Pendular exercises were conducted after each Quadriceps strengthening, in between isometrics and isotonics.The three outcome measures First Swing Excursion, Number Of Oscillations and Duration of Oscillations were analysed before and after Quadriceps strengthening. Pre and Post test was conducted.

The FSE in some of the CP children involved in the study showed a slight increase which indicates the increase in the degree of range of motion during post test. As a result, it can be stated that the spasticity can be decreased slightly after Quadriceps strengthening. The FSE has increased from 77.17 degree of ROM in pre test to 78.04 degree ROM in the post test showing the improvement. So when the FSE increases every time during post test, range of motion tends to improve which ultimately leads to decrease in spasticity.

When the range of motion of FSE increases during post test, the subsequent outcome measure which is the number of oscillations also increases during post test. The NoOS has increased from 3.93 in pre test to 4.67 in the post test showing the improvement. From the post test, it was evident that FSE and NoOS are directly proportional. It ultimately states that when FSE increases during post test, spasticity decreases. As a result of decreased spasticity, it becomes easier for the cerebral palsy children involved in the study, to increase the number of pendular exercises and thereby increases the number of oscillations.

The post test gives a clear picture that FSE and NoOS are directly proportional, but however it is, FSE and NoOS with DOS are inversely related. This is due to the fact when FSE increases during post test, NoOS also increases and the patients who are the cerebral palsy children involved in the study are able to perform more number of oscillations within limited number of DOS which remains stagnant without any increase or decrease.

In most of the cerebral palsy children involved in the study, there showed an increase in FSE and NoOS, but the DOS was neither increased nor decreased and it is maintained in the same level.

In contrary to the null hypothesis which was rejected, there were significant changes in spasticity during post test as per alternate hypothesis which was proved to be true. Although there is no marked improvement, spasticity has decreased to a certain extent after post test preventing the exaggeration of spasticity.

However it is, analysis of the post test of all the cerebral palsy children involved in the study revealed that there were no deteriorating effects of Quadriceps strengthening on spasticity in children with spastic diplegic cerebral palsy.

CONCLUSION

.

The results of this study do not support the premise that Quadriceps femoris strengthening exercises with maximum efforts increase spasticity in children with Cerebral palsy based on the outcome measures.These results, considered along with the results of other studies that have demonstrated improvements in force production in individuals with CP, suggest that there are no detrimental effects associated with muscle strengthening programs. Results may promote the use of strengthening exercises in children with CP where muscle weakness may contribute to functional problems.

LIMITATIONS AND RECOMMENDATIONS

LIMITATIONS

➢ The subjects involved in study were of a particular age group i.e below 10 years

➢ The subjects were less

➢ Duration of study was short

RECOMMENDATIONS

➢ The study can include age group of above 14 years

➢ The study can include adolescent cp cases.

➢ The study can be conducted to study a greater improvement in ROM after strengthening exercise

➢ The study can be conducted to study about improvement in gait pattern after strengthening exercise

➢ The number of subjects included in the study can be more.

➢ The study can be conducted with longer duration

REFERENCES

1. Mutch L, Alberman E, Hagberg B, et al. Cerebral palsy epidemiology: where are we now and where are we going? Dev Med Child Neurol. 1992;34(6):547–51. [PubMed]

2. Michael RB. Management of spasticity. Age Ageing. 1998;27(2):239–45. [PubMed]

3. Goldstein EM. Spasticity management: an overview. J Child Neurol. 2001;16(1):16–23. [PubMed]

4. Tilton AH. Management of spasticity in children with cerebral palsy. Semin Pediatr Neurol. 2004;11(1):58–65. [PubMed]

5. Matthews DJ, Balaban B. Management of spasticity in children with cerebral palsy. Acta Orthop Traumatol Turc. 2009;43(2):81–6. [PubMed]

6. Chan NNC. Physiotherapy in Spasticity Management for Children with Cerebral Palsy. Hong KongMed Bulletin. 2011;16(7):24–6.

7. Gage J, Gormley Jr M, Krach L, et al. Managing spasticity in children with cerebral palsy requires a team approach. a pediatric perspective. Gillette Children Spatiality Health Care. 2004;13(3)

8. Rassafiani M, Sahaf R. Hypertonicity in children with cerebral palsy: a new perspective. IRJ. 2011;9(0):66–74.

9. Khalid AM, Sabahat AW. Management of spastic cerebral palsy in the UAE: An overview. ACNR. 2009;9(2):30–2

10. Fowler EG,Ho TW, Nwigwe AI, Dorey F. The effect of quadriceps femoris muscle strengthening exercises on spasticity in children with cerebral palsy *Phys Ther.* 2001;81:1215–1223.

11. Bobath K. *A Neurophysiological Basis for the Treatment of Cerebral Palsy.* 2nd ed. London, England: William Heinemann Medical Books Ltd,1980 .

12. Horak FB. Assumptions underlying motor control for neurologic rehabilitation. In: Lister MJ, eds. *Contemporary Management of Motor Control Problems. Proceedings of the II STEP Conference.* Alexandria, Va: Foundation for Physical Therapy,1991 :11–27.

13. Healy A. Two methods of weight-training for children with spastic type   of cerebral palsy. *Res Q.*1958; 29:389–395.

14. Damiano DL, Kelly LE, Vaughn CL. Effects of quadriceps femoris muscle strengthening on crouch gait in children with spastic diplegia. *Phys Ther.*1995; 75:658–671.

15. Damiano DL, Vaughan CL, Abel MF. Muscle response to heavy resistance exercise in children with spastic cerebral palsy. *Dev Med Child Neurol.*1995; 37:731–739.

16. McCubbin JA, Shasby GB. Effects of isokinetic exercise on adolescents with cerebral palsy. *Adapted Physical Activity Quarterly.*1985; 2:56–64.

17. MacPhail HEA, Kramer JF. Effect of isokinetic strength-training on functional ability and walking efficiency in adolescents with cerebral palsy. *Dev Med Child Neurol.*1995; 37:763–775.

18. Hovart M. Effects of a progressive resistance training program on an individual with spastic cerebral palsy. *American Corrective Therapy Journal.*1987; 41:7–11.

19. Bohannon RW, Smith MB. Interrater reliability of a modified Ashworth scale of muscle spasticity. *Phys Ther.*1987; 67:206–207.

20. Lance JW. Symposium synopsis. In: Feldman RG, Young RR, Koella WP, eds. *Spasticity: Disordered Motor Control.* Chicago, Ill: Year Book Medical,1980 :485–494.

21. Price R. Mechanical spasticity evaluation techniques. *Physical and Rehabilitation Medicine.*1990; 2:65–73.

22. Robinson CJ, Kett NA, Bolam JM. Spasticity in spinal cord injured patients, 2: initial measures and long-term effects of surface electrical stimulation. *Arch Phys Med Rehabil.*1988; 69:862–868.

23. Brar SP, Smith MB, Nelson LM, et al. Evaluation of treatment protocols on minimal to moderate spasticity in multiple sclerosis. *Arch Phys Med Rehabil.*1991; 72:186–189.

25.Wartenberg R. Pendulousness of the legs as a diagnostic test. *Neurology.*1951; 1:18–24.

26. Bohannon RW. Variability and reliability of the pendulum test for spasticity using a Cybex II isokinetic dynamometer. *Phys Ther*.1987; 67:659–661.

27. Fowler EG, Nwigwe AI, Ho TW. Sensitivity of the pendulum test for assessing spasticity in persons with cerebral palsy. *Dev Med Child Neurol*.2000; 42:182–189.

28. Peacock WJ, Staudt LA. Functional outcomes following selective posterior rhizotomy in children with cerebral palsy. *J Neurosurg*.1991; 74:380–385.

29. Bajd T, Bowman B. Testing and modelling of spasticity. *J Biomed Eng*.1982; 4:90–96

30. Brown RA, Lawson DA, Leslie GC, Part NJ. Observations on the applicability of the Wartenberg pendulum test to healthy, elderly subjects. *J Neurol Neurosurg Psychiatry*.1988; 51:1171–1177.[

31. Bobath B. *Adult Hemiplegia: Evaluation and Treatment*. 2nd ed. London, England: William Heinemann Medical Books Ltd,1978 .

32. Bobath K. *The Motor Deficits in Patients With Cerebral Palsy. Clinics in Developmental Medicine, No. 23*. Philadelphia, Pa: JB Lippincott Co,1966 .

33. Gowland CA, deBruin H, Basmajian JV, et al. Agonist and antagonist activity during voluntary upper-limb movement in patients with stroke. *Phys Ther*.1992; 72:624–633

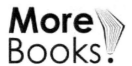

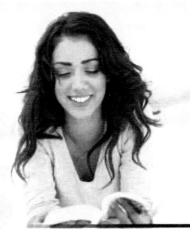

I want morebooks!

Buy your books fast and straightforward online - at one of world's
fastest growing online book stores! Environmentally sound due to
Print-on-Demand technologies.

Buy your books online at
www.morebooks.shop

Kaufen Sie Ihre Bücher schnell und unkompliziert online – auf einer
der am schnellsten wachsenden Buchhandelsplattformen weltweit!
Dank Print-On-Demand umwelt- und ressourcenschonend produzi
ert.

Bücher schneller online kaufen
www.morebooks.shop

KS OmniScriptum Publishing
Brivibas gatve 197
LV-1039 Riga, Latvia   info@omniscriptum.com   OMNIScriptum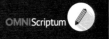
Telefax: +371 686 204 55   www.omniscriptum.com

MIX
Papier aus verantwortungsvollen Quellen
Paper from responsible sources
FSC® C105338
FSC
www.fsc.org

Printed by Books on Demand GmbH, Norderstedt / Germany